DISABLE

Survival Guide

By Tim Patten

ISBN-13:
978-1724403254

ISBN-10:
1724403257

Worldwide Copyright © 2018, Timothy G. Patten. Writers Guild Registered. All rights reserved. No part of this book may be reproduced or transmitted in any form or by any means, electronic or mechanical, including photocopying, recording or by any information storage and retrieval system, without permission of the author, except for the inclusion of brief quotations in a review.

DISABLED AND UNABLE TO WORK

Now What?

SURVIVAL GUIDE

How to Navigate your Disability Claim and Qualify for Insurer's Pay Checks

Tim Patten

DISCLOSURE

The content of this book is not a substitute for professional representation by a legal, disability, psychological, medical, or financial specialist. Under no circumstances will the author, its principals, or any of its affiliates, or any public adjuster, lawyer or advisor listed here, be responsible for (1) any information contained in or omitted from this content, (2) any person's reliance on any such information, whether or not the information is correct, current or complete, (3) any person's satisfaction with any financial service, lawyer or advisor, whether relating to their competence, diligence or otherwise, whether or not they are an advertiser on this site, (4) the results of any advice given by or representation from any public adjuster, specialist, lawyer or advisor, (5) the financial consequence of any investment made by the reader (5) the consequence of any action you or any other person takes or fails to take, whether or not based on information provided by or as a result of the use of this book.

All people, characters, company names and insurance companies in this book are fictionalized in order to protect identities. The book is not describing any single company's business procedures. The outline and characters are loosely based on the lives of American's that have been tormented by disability and their Long-Term Disability insurers. Any likeness between the fictionalized composite characters in this book and any one person's real life are unintentional and entirely circumstantial.

INTRODUCTION

Each year, more than 2.2 million Americans experience an accident, injury or illness that temporarily or permanently ends their ability to work, threatens their livelihoods, and forces them to file a long-term disability claim. Out of all those who apply, only 3 % will ever receive disability payments. The other 97 % will never see a penny, as their claims will be rejected. How can you make sure this doesn't happen to you?

The insurance company investigating your claim will work to protect your former employer by seeking out loopholes and using every trick in the book to disqualify your claim. While the journey ahead is riddled with potential pitfalls, this book will be your closest ally, providing survival tips, warnings, and examples of real case scenarios. to empower and guide you as you navigate the claim's process. It will help you with the practical, as well as, the spiritual aspects of your journey to rediscover life's meaning and purpose, after the devastation of disability. This easy-to-follow guide will walk you through the steps of submitting your claim, qualifying for disability pay, and ultimately learning to thrive in this new chapter of your life.

"How to Navigate your Disability Claim and Qualify for Insurer's Pay Checks"

Contents

Chapter 1	Disability and Trauma
Chapter 2	Your Doctor and Qualifying for Benefits
Chapter 3	Elsie Moore Files a Disability Claim
Chapter 4	Plan Your Exit from Work
Chapter 5	Mental Health
Chapter 6	Gloria Carter's First Week Homebound
Chapter 7	Your Physical Health
Chapter 8	Gloria's 11th Week Homebound
Chapter 9	Should I Get a Lawyer?
Chapter 10	Insurance Company Paranoia
Chapter 11	Get Your House in Order
Chapter 12	The Morning Mail
Chapter 13	More Details
Chapter 14	The COBRA Process and Options
Chapter 15	Selling Your Life Insurance
Chapter 16	An Inspector Calls
Chapter 17	What's Next Financially
Chapter 18	Finding Your Meaningful Purpose

Chapter 1
Disability and Trauma

You are now seriously injured or ill and have or will file a claim for benefits under your employer's disability insurance policy. This form of coverage provides those who are unable to work with monthly payments that typically represent a %, perhaps 50% or more, of what they made while they were working. In doing so, you will be seeking to join some 19 % of Americans, or 60 million people, who are in similar circumstances; disabled and unable to work.

Depending on the types of plan and other issues being covered, you may have or will file a claim for either a **short** or **long-term** disability payments. Major insurance providers of this type of coverage, which is typically offered through employers (though individuals can also purchase it directly from many of the companies involved), such as **Aflac, Unum, Cigna, Liberty Mutual, MetLife, and Aetna**.

Although clearly similar, this type of coverage is separate and distinct from that which is available through the Federal Social Security Disability program. In many respects, private disability benefits are viewed as a more viable supplement to the meager benefits available through the government-run program.

At the beginning of 2015, for instance, Social Security paid an average disability benefit of $1,165 per month, which was barely enough to keep a beneficiary above the 2015 poverty level of $11,770 per year, for a single person.

Given that, it is no surprise that many of those who have chosen to sign up for private disability insurance did whatever they could to keep their policies going, and to avoid being left in the lurch, if or when misfortune struck and they couldn't work.

Unfortunately, the promises that many disability insurers made about what policyholders would get in the event of a claim, have become increasingly empty. Over time, these insurers have simply failed to honor most of their obligations.

This book is not intended to single out any of these insurers, however. Rather, it is intended to discuss what has occurred in the industry more broadly and how that can affect someone like you, who are confronting the challenge of getting what is owed. Nevertheless, it's worth pointing out that the reviews posted online from disability insurance policyholders tend to be fairly abysmal, with verified ratings averaging around *one* out of a possible *five* stars.

Indeed, customers regularly accuse these companies of any number of deceptive or unethical practices, ranging from delaying authorizations and required payments to simply denying claims for the wrong reasons, often nitpicking on dates and doctor's notes. Increasingly, they pepper those making claims, with repeated requests for additional medical evidence of a disability, even if it has already been proved to a reasonable standard. The result is that **70% of you will not be paid back and awarded your disability pay!**

With this in mind, you will need to be prepared and ready for action. You must empower yourself for what will likely prove to be a challenging and at times, exhausting experience. You will also need to fully understand the various steps that will be required to navigate the claim process and get what is owed, allowing you to carry on living with your disability without being left impoverished, or in a state of nagging despair.

Initially, this book discusses the emotional trauma you'll likely experience even before you begin the process. Subsequent chapters will offer survival tips and highlight warnings you'll need to pay attention to. Some are dire. They are not intended to frighten, but to harden you and guide you through the practical realities of adjusting to your new job of "working your disability."

You may need to dedicate considerable time and energy each day, possibly for months, to labor through your claim.

For a newly disabled person, the road to getting what you are rightly owed is typically full of potholes, sharp turns, and bridges that may collapse, seemingly out of the blue. In fact, making your insurance company live up to its obligations may be one of the most difficult things you have ever endured, which is saying something. Worse still, you may find you are often on your own when it comes to avoiding the booby traps that can send your potential disability checks into the trash bin.

You have been left alone inside the worst thunderstorm of your life. You are vulnerable to the sheets of torrential rains and raw gusting winds. Your body is buffeted back and forth. What is on the horizon?

This book can make it easier. It can help strengthen your resolve and raise your awareness in a way that will allow you to see and step over each and every step, crack, pothole, and crevice along the way. Only by gaining an understanding beforehand of the pitfalls you will invariably face, and the slings and arrows the insurance companies will inevitably send your way, can you get to the place where you deserve to be.

The Hidden Dark Side

Before you became disabled, you were most likely blind to a reality that is hidden behind shadows, and inside closed attics. Now, though, your incapacity has turned a spotlight on the underworld of life on disability. At first, you'll have trouble wrapping your mind around the meaninglessness associated with not being able to work. Combined with the many obstacles you'll face; this will likely leave you feeling that your self-worth has reached its lowest point and that your life is basically over.

It will take time for your inner self to come to terms with the fact that a disease or injury has taken away your ability to work, and the freedom to make an honest living and to provide a value of some kind. For most of us, our conscious minds have spent a lifetime preparing for work, seeking it out, and being productive. Much of our history, education, and relationships have been tied in some way, to such activity.

In fact, if you are like many people, you may have strived long and hard for recognition, pay raises, and the rewards that only come from having a job or running a business. For us men, in particular, it has generally been the case that we closely identify "who we are" with our job or career. With that in mind, you might easily find yourself in a state of denial and take all sorts of pains to try to return to rewarding work, however difficult or implausible that may be in your current state.

Prepare for Anxiety

In reality, you should not be surprised to feel as if your entire world and sense of value have been shattered into little bits, and that any instinctual desires you might have had, need to be reoriented or redesigned from scratch. As with many major life events, you may need considerable time, perhaps a year or more, just to come to terms with your new world order and become attuned to your body and mind's changing rhythms and actions.

More than likely, you'll be shocked at what you'll discover. You'll realize that you have been living in two universes. While you have been familiar with the techniques and methods on how able-bodied people interact with the world, you will now see another dark place where people cannot do many things, including paying the bills or keeping a home running smoothly. You are now at the place where those who cannot work, or fully contribute the resources needed for survival.

Think about the dreams you might have had, whether about financial success or new positions, responsibilities, and raises. Did you envision retirement on a desert island? Did you have a desire to be the best at your job, or to climb the economic ladder to its highest rungs? Did your aspirations include exciting vacation travels to exotic destinations with the love of your life?

Now, though, matters have changed for the worse. These hopeful images have suddenly been shorn into bits and shards, turning from exciting ambitions to sudden hopelessness, and the feeling that they may never be achieved. Under such circumstances, it is only natural that you might begin to find yourself immersed and wallowing in feelings of *malaise and anxiety.*

Prepare for Melancholy and Depression

Now that you are disabled, the act of simply existing can seem grim and morose, as if you have fallen into a darkly terrifying abyss, with no means of righting yourself as you descend to its depths. You can no longer work to improve your world. Most, if not all, of the methods and techniques that were once so familiar to you as you moved your non-disabled self toward whatever objective you might have set out to achieve, are no longer valid.

At this point, you will need to develop new tools and perspectives. You will need to educate yourself, most likely, with some assistance, about how to navigate the turbulent and rough waters that lay ahead. You will have to adapt to a myriad of new challenges, most of which you will not have even been aware of before. You will need to tailor a lifestyle that can help you survive and thrive in the face of an existence that your old life has left you well unprepared for.

Making matters worse, you will be constantly reminded of what might have been when you were able to work and bring home the bacon. Everything you see on television or online will make it clear what you can no longer afford. Every advertisement, especially those aimed at people living upwardly mobile lives, will reinforce the notion that your budget has become a barrier. Every story you read or hear will trigger a longing for ambitions and dreams you once held deep. All of this can lead to *melancholy and depression.*

Prepare for Potential Substance Abuse

Many of us enjoy the uninhibited and relaxing sensitivities associated with having a beer – or perhaps, several beers. Unfortunately, the evidence suggests that no small number of people, especially males, tend to overconsume and become addicted to mind-altering substances after being forced out of work because of disability.

It's not hard to see that those who don't work or have the responsibilities of a job might go this way out of boredom. In addition, given the pain, and stress, and other challenges that many disabled individuals have to deal with, it is not surprising at all that at least, some will imbibe more than usual, to cope. Nevertheless, while the need to hide or escape from reality might seem like an answer, *it is not really a viable solution.*

The sad truth is that one beer or cocktail can easily become two, and then, turn into many more, over the course of time. Eventually, getting sloshed can evolve from a once-a-week activity to a daily routine. In the end, it can quickly evolve into a costly physical addiction, where the body needs the substance every day, simply to feel normal. Below are some signs that suggest a problem is brewing (so to speak):

- You've passed out after drinking on one occasion or another.
- You find that a drunken state unexpectedly creeps up on you.
- You say and do foolish things that are not really funny to others.
- Your ability to walk and function normally becomes noticeably impaired.
- You become increasingly angry, or critical toward friends and family.
- Those who are closest to you begin to point out unwelcome personality changes.
- You frequently swallow aspirins, pain pills, or other drugs, in an effort to get a better sleep.
- You can't wait to have that first drink of the day.

Alcohol isn't the only substance that people use for self-medication, of course. Another popular remedy is marijuana – weed. This plant has become more widely available amid a nationwide push for decriminalization. Although indications of overuse are somewhat similar to those associated with alcohol, weed does not appear to create a physical addiction. Rather, it fosters more of a psychological need, where the brain craves the sensation of being high.

Other products that are being abused in this way include prescription painkillers' such as opioids. In fact, this category of prescription drugs appears to have become a major gateway to deadly addictions that claim the lives of more than 60,000 people each year.

But substances designed to dull pain aren't the only ones being used as a means of escape. Other examples include barbiturates, which are nonselective central nervous system depressants that were once a mainstay for sedating patients or inducing sleep. More recently, these have been replaced by benzodiazepines, such as Valium (Diazepam) and Ativan (Lorazepam), which are intended to treat anxiety and are supposedly, less likely, to cause physical dependence and severe withdrawal.

As with alcohol, there are various markers that can signal that a pain remedy or other treatment has turned into something else, including the following:

- You take a pill every time you feel frustrated or headachy.
- You willingly consume more medication than prescribed.
- You burn crushed pills on tin foil to sniff the vapor.
- You become more forgetful or nap or fall asleep at odd times.
- You have ringing in your ears, blurred vision, or constricted pupils.
- Your mouth feels numb to the touch, or your fingers tremble inexplicably.
- Your heartbeat feels low or you experience lightheadedness or confusion.
- You have hardened stools or constipation.

If you find that you are in a troubling situation with regard to alcohol, weed, pills or any other mind-altering substances, the good news is that there are strategies you can use that can help you turn the tide without needing to reach out for the expensive rehabilitation provided by medical professionals. Regardless, it is imperative that you remain mindful of the threat of *substance abuse*.

Prepare for Possible Social Isolation

Another downside of being disabled is the prospect of reduced contact with other people and co-workers. At some point, you'll stop seeing the many individuals you saw every day on the way to the job, at work, and on the way home. You may never see most, if not all, of the co-workers or customers you might previously have mingled with on a regular basis. You won't run into others, whether known or unknown while picking up coffee or buying groceries. Separated from the sorts of interactions that many take for granted, your world may become very small, and you may experience *social isolation*.

Prepare for Possible Suicide

One particularly serious risk for those who have been left unable to do what they used to do is the potential for self-harm. For middle-aged white men, in particular, being forced to leave work because of disability can feel shameful and traumatic, leading to despair, depression, and, in no small number of cases, suicide.

While most people will likely feel seriously affected, the fact that men have long been seen as the breadwinners, which has become integral to who they are, can have a devastating impact.

Men have also been viewed as the "Mr. Fixits," in charge of repairing leaking pipes, or dealing with any other mechanical issues on behalf of their families, and society at large. They are likely to be stolid in the face of any threats or challenges that life may throw at them, and to attend to the numerous emotional grievances of a partner or child – in other words, they represent the shoulder for everyone else to cry on.

When things change, and you suddenly feel that you've become a burden to others, or that the identity they once had no longer exists, it can foster all sorts of dark and desperate thoughts. Add that to the feelings of unfamiliarity and impotence that can arise when roles are reversed, or when someone feels unable to cope with a dramatic change in their lives, and it can easily lead to someone considering the ultimate escape: *suicide*.

Potential Dismantled Families

Even if things don't reach that point, the impact can be far-reaching. When someone who has played a vital role in a family or other such relationship can no longer do so, it can cause havoc, and undermine existing household structures. Teens and twenty-somethings may be asked to go to work and pay rent or help with living expenses. Other family members may be asked to step up and find a new or better job – or a second one – and work longer hours, creating numerous strains.

And even if it doesn't mean somebody has to go out and bring in more cash, most, if not all, members of the household will likely have to take on extra responsibilities. Regardless of what gender they are, they may have to handle roles and chores that they don't want to do or are not familiar with, including helping the person who is disabled to manage basic personal and bodily functions. Such changes will likely boost the degree of stress, conflict, and arguments, in the household.

Sadly, depending on the age of those involved and the financial resources that are available, some of the non-disabled members could simply decide to check out. Some women view men as utilities; only useful if they produce regular paychecks, reflecting a hypergamy that is pervasive in our society.

Should a wife, for example, decide that there is no future in a relationship with a disabled spouse? It could easily lead to disruption and pain. In sum, *disabilities can splinter relationships, families, and even friendships into many little pieces.*

Conclusion

Still, even with all the challenges listed in this chapter, your new life on disability does not have to mean the end of the world, as you know it. Rather, it should be seen as a radical transformation of what living means to you. You are hunched over in the midst of a terrorizing storm; now is the time you must learn to dance against the turbulence. Your unfolding destiny will entail suffering, but you will also have opportunities to learn and experience great personal triumphs. You can and will meet the challenges and manage them with personal grace. As you go through the experience, you will become someone you never thought about before: a warrior of the battle with disease and health, overcoming all obstacles.

Chapter 2
Your Doctor and Qualifying for Benefits

If you are disabled, your primary care doctor is clearly important when it comes to looking after your health and other needs. However, when it comes to getting the disability benefits you are entitled to, she (or he) is the gatekeeper. Quite simply, without their support, you will never qualify.

In fact, it is in your absolute best interest to develop a long and trustworthy relationship with this medical professional, who will effectively be your golden key throughout the process. You will need to ensure they are the main decision maker with respect to your health, treatment options, and documentation of your health status.

This may not be as easy as it sounds. Nowadays, doctors are forced by insurance rules and the realities of the healthcare marketplace, to turn their patient's visits around every nine to fifteen minutes. This means that the quality time you spend with your physician may be very limited. You probably won't be able to learn enough during your interactions with them, at a time when their advice is vitally important.

The fact is that, while the doctor may not literally be your best friend or a member of the family, in many ways, they will be playing that role. For one thing, after probing and prodding virtually every inch of you, they will likely know more about you physically than most other people, including your partner or mother.

In reality, if you treat your visits with your doctor the way you should, you'll likely end up having frank discussions about sensitive or embarrassing topics. You'll need to be able to mention, for example, a rash on your scrotum, or a lump inside your rectum. For the doctor to be the advocate you will need going forward, it is important to establish a baseline measure of trust.

If you have a phobia of doctors or the healthcare system more generally, it's a good bet that your disability will cure those fears because you will now be visiting clinics and hospitals on a regular basis. You will also be seeing your primary doctor a lot. Either way, you should be seeking to get the most out of these visits, both in terms of the diagnoses and treatments you receive, and your understanding of what is going on. **To do this, you should take copious notes before each visit; noting the things you don't understand or need to know.**

Medical Documentation

It's not just you, of course, who should be recording any relevant information. You may, for instance, visit a variety of physicians or mental health professionals to treat your illness. The latter is not uncommon when it comes to people suffering from chronic illness; many are also plagued by anguish and depression. It is in your interest to ensure that all of these encounters, and any relevant evidence is properly documented in the official records.

The fact is that while many insurance companies won't authorize disability payouts based solely on psychological or substance abuse issues, they may make for compelling, additional evidence, when taken together with other data that details your inability to work.

Activities of Daily Living Documentation

One common mistake that claimants often make is focusing solely on their diagnosis. Based on this sort of "tunnel vision" thinking, they may assume that such a finding automatically confirms they are disabled and entitled to benefits. This is especially true of people suffering from such disorders as fibromyalgia and chronic fatigue syndrome.

In reality, when a medical professional makes a diagnosis that a physical or psychological condition prevents you from working, that is only the beginning rather than the end of the data needed in a claim process. After that, the next stage is to set it all down on paper, fully documenting every aspect of your disability. Needless to say, all your statements must be accurate and complete, and they must make it clear that what you are going through has had a major impact on your life.

Take chronic pain and fatigue, for example. It is critical that you distinguish why these symptoms are different from what an average person might experience on any given day. If you say, "I'm in pain and fatigued," that doesn't explain very much. Why? From time to time, we all experience some measure of pain or fatigue. All you are really saying with that sort of statement, is that you are a normal human being.

However, if you tell your doctor, "I am unable to function, wash dishes and prepare food, as I experience severe daily pain and exhausting fatigue, lasting most of the day without relief," or "I am unable to dress and bathe myself three days per week due to migraine headaches that last all day, even with medication," now, you've given the doctor – who is considered an impartial mediator – a better picture of why your symptoms are so debilitating, and why you should be seen as disabled.

For the most part, you generally want to provide information based on what the situation is like, with respect to your worst days, not your good days. Below are some comparative statements that show the ways in which your symptoms and experience should be presented:

Do not say: "I must sit to prepare meals."
Do say: "I can no longer stand at the kitchen counter, in order to prepare for meals."

Do not say: "I shop for myself."
Do say: "I buy only a few items at a time. I can't carry many bags, and more importantly, I can't put away a lot of groceries when I get home. I can't spend a lot of time in the store, either, so I have to keep making many short trips."

Do not say: "I do laundry."
Do say: "I can do only one load of laundry at a time, although I used to do all of it at once. I cannot put away the clean clothes on the same day that I do the laundry. That is now a task for another day. I no longer keep up with the laundry, since I have to wait for a time when I feel up to the task, and those good days are not necessarily when I need clean clothes."

Do not say: "I can't make my own meals."
Do say: "I no longer make complete meals, and no longer invite guests for dinner. I eat simpler foods so that I don't need to spend as much time as I used to, in preparing meals. Sometimes, I need to rest before I can finish making something to eat."

As a rule, if you are making the argument that you are totally disabled, you'll need to have plenty of evidence in your charts that you're unable to perform activities of daily living when the insurer reviews your case over necessary time-frames. What are these activities? The following table sets out what they are according to the healthcare community:

Activities of Daily Living (ADL)

ADL Function	Independent	Needs Help	Dependent	Cannot Do
Bathing				
Dressing				
Grooming				
Mouth care				
Toileting				
Transferring bed/chair				
Walking				
Climbing stairs				
Eating				

Conclusion

As you likely have already realized, your disability and your inability to work create a maelstrom of impediments that surround you. In some respects, you are at the vortex of a dangerous storm, one that may be a threat to your existence.

But life cannot be focused on changing the bad weather, which comes whether you like it or not. It is about learning to dance through the tornadoes and grab hold of new opportunities barely visible in between the howling winds, wet chills, and blinding flashes of lightning. One dance partner you must hold tight to is your doctor.

In the next chapter, you will meet Elsie Moore, a kind and giving person, who assumed her friends at work had her best interests in mind.

Chapter 3
Elsie Moore Files a Disability Claim

Elsie Moore chirped, "Welcome to The EveryDayGrocer!" It required all of her energy to feign a cheerful grin.

"Elsie, you been draggin' for months," Carol said. "You're supposed to be a happy face. What's wrong?"

Elsie finished ringing up the customer's groceries. "Thank you for shopping at The EveryDayGrocer!" She turned to Carol and said, "I'm just so tired all the time. These days, I can't really be bothered to cook. I've been eating easy food ever since Frank passed away." Her husband had contracted black lung after many years in the coal industry.

"He's been gone for a good two years," Carol said gently. "Don't you think it's about time you got checked out? I know a good doctor right here in Rock Hill. I'll give you his number."

Elsie shrugged. "Fine—I'll tell you. I know what it is. They found it quite late, but I've known for a while. I just don't like to make a fuss about it. Back when I was pregnant with Tommy, my doctor told me I have lupus."

"Never heard of such a thing."

"It's not all that rare. It's a chronic disease affecting my immune system. It causes pain, fatigue, and tissue damage all throughout my body."

"Isn't there anything you can take for it?"

"I've been prescribed some pain medications and treatments that will slow the organ damage. But it's unlikely the symptoms will ever completely disappear."

"Does Human Resources know?"

"I told Jeannie in HR on my first day. And recently, when I took more sick days than usual, she offered to help me out by reducing some of my responsibilities. She has been so nice. So yeah, I signed for a small rearrangement."

Carol nodded. "Jeanie's great. I love working here. We're so lucky. We have great benefits."

"And I've needed them more than ever, with Frank gone." Elsie still felt the sting of disbelief whenever she acknowledged his absence. She frowned. "But I don't know how much longer I can keep working. It's time I filed for disability."

"Only you can say what's best for you."

"I called Jeannie last week, and I'll sign the forms when they come in. I guess I'll be leaving work soon."

"I'll miss you, Elsie. Enjoy your retirement!"

"Thank you, Carol. I'll miss you too."

A week later, Elsie and her doctor filled out the forms. She's expected to receive 60 % of her $28K annual salary, which would come to around $20K, paid in monthly instalments. She would be able to maintain her simple lifestyle in the little town of Rock Hill. Tommy, her only child, had already grown up and moved out. She would be able to hire a home health worker to come by every week, bring her groceries, do her laundry, run her errands, and clean up her house. When she received the insurance company's letter, she eagerly opened it.

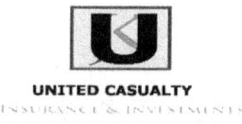

UNITED CASUALTY
INSURANCE & INVESTMENTS

1 5 9 856
info@jacksonia....om
www.jacks...kennedy.com
P.O. Box 3˙   3, hill street, NY

Claimant:	Elsie Mae Moore	Date:	01/02/2010
Case#:	900122	SSNO:	XXX-XX-2908
Claim:	000771	Emp:	Grocers

Dear Mrs. Elsie Mae Moore,

We've reviewed your ongoing claim for long-term disability benefits. Our medical examiner has found there is no policy that covers your current part-time position. Your claim is now closed as of the date of this notification letter.

Dr. Ben Boultwood
Medical Claims Examiner
United Casualty Insurance Company

Elsie's heart skipped a beat. She had not seen this coming. Jeannie had been so reassuring. Anxiety surged through her body with bone-crushing pressure. Was there any way to fight this? She couldn't afford a lawyer. How would she survive? To whom could she turn? An image of her beloved Frank appeared in a fog, surrounded by white light.

Her heart continued to race, as she tried to juggle her monthly bills in a vain attempt to stay within her Social Security budget of $1700 each month. With her fist pressed against her face, she calculated the cost of her medications and a home health worker. There wasn't enough money to cover both. She wondered whether she could do her own shopping and laundry. The answer was no. She rubbed the center of her forehead for a few minutes, before slipping a Valium into her mouth.

Within four months, she had maxed out all of her credit cards to cover doctor visits and medications. She felt as though, her debt was an inescapable burden that would plague her for the rest of her days on Earth.

Conclusion

Elsie Moore discovered that the primary objective of the Human Resources department is to reduce the organization's claims costs.

Human Resources serves the company rather than its employees. This book reveals to you, the reader, many of the methods used by HR departments and the disability insurer to manipulate outcomes so that you'll be better prepared to do battle when the time comes.

Chapter 4
Plan Your Exit from Work

You're employed full-time, and a serious injury or an illness is pushing you ever closer, to the point at which it will become impossible for you to continue working. This is a critical step in your disability journey when the key figures in your organization—including your boss and the Human Resources department—are no longer aligned with you. They have become your opponents. Together, they will employ every weapon in their arsenal, to oppose you and your claim.

Cast your mind back and try to remember your employer's benefits handbook. It may be a distant memory, but you might remember that it promised that if you became disabled, they had promised to pay 50 % (or a higher %) of your salary until you reach the age of sixty-five.

While this sounds simple enough, as Elsie Moore discovered in the previous chapter, many loopholes and obstacles stand in the way of your organization's financial fulfillment of those promises. Orchestrating your exit from your full-time job is *the most important thing* in your life right now. A well-planned exit will help you to ensure the steps to a decent financial future.

Your chance for future wellness depends on your ability to hold on to the finances obtained, and cash in on insurance promises.

For this reason, you should **never** mention to anyone, especially not to those in management, that you plan to take short-term or long-term leave from your job.

In the interests of being honest and open, you may have already told the company about your plan to leave work. The moment you tell Human Resources or your boss you are unable to work and want to file for the company disability plan, you have ceased to be a valued employee. You have become a cost or business liability that must be circumvented, and your company will do everything within its power, to avoid fulfilling its financial responsibility to you.

Chronic Illness vs. Injury or Accident

An employee with a chronic medical condition will often make a gradual progression towards eventual disability. A person in these circumstances does not get up one day, realize that he or she is sick, and then, leave on disability. Instead, a worker might be able to continue working for many years with little or no outward sign of illness. While they may appear to be in full health, their work performance or attendance may begin to decline, as they take intermittent sick days or leave days for doctor visits and exhibit a lack of strength or stamina. These workers are candidates for losing their full-time job, along with all their benefits. Therefore, they must plan ahead.

How Organizations Disrupt Disability Claims

Method 1: Elsie Moore's experience of sharing her health status typifies how those in management or HR will offer to lower your work stress by working out a lighter schedule. While this may be construed as an act of sympathy, they are actually *asking you to sign off on subtle or gradual changes*. The reality is that you will be transferred to part-time employment, in which all your full-time benefits, including disability insurance, are no longer available.

It may come as a surprise that Human Resources or your boss will turn against you. For many companies, when an employee files a disability claim, reducing the cost often takes priority over the humane treatment of the (soon to be former) employee. Your organization and the insurance company may try to trick you into voluntarily surrendering these financial benefits. In many instances, employees lose their financial disability benefits because they are slow to recognize what's happening to their health and delay making their claim for disability pay.

Method 2: Once your organization knows you are going to claim disability, it may *eliminate your position* before your disability claim paperwork has been processed. The organization can then, reject your disability claim, on the grounds that your position has been closed.

When it comes to disrupting your claim, the company has the upper hand. As an illness or injury gradually depletes an employee's productive powers, the person will often be in denial about what's happening. They will tell themselves: *This is just a temporary setback. I'll get better soon. I'm really not that sick.* This is natural. Productive people don't want to dwell on negative thoughts. The brain has been trained to defend the body by dwelling on positive thoughts. Be honest with yourself about the condition of your health. Be realistic about your limitations.

Method 3: A company can *transfer or change your position* by offering much lower pay or moving you to another physical location, thus, placing obstacles in the way of the disability pay you might be awarded.

Companies have a set of diverse and ingenious techniques to derail your disability claim process. Employers will appear to be sympathetic to your plight. It's likely you'll be offered a new position. They might craft a less strenuous position just for you. That sounds good, but it may be a strategic move. This new position might have a classification other than full-time. It may be a position exempt from disability insurance. Remember, you don't have the legal insurance policy to read. Only your employer's HR staff knows the policy's loopholes and details.

Who knows how long your new, low-stress position will stay funded by the company? You may come in one day to find it has been dropped. You could find a pink slip, severance pay, and legal forms ready for you to sign. You'll not be entitled to any disability insurance benefits.

Method 4: Most companies will require you to first file a short-term disability claim, which typically covers only three to six months. *Once the short-term benefits expire, the long-term disability is ignored*, and those benefits are not claimed within an efficient time frame. Long-term insurance will promise to pay out between 50 and 70 % of your salary. Typically, policies will pay you until the age of sixty-five, or for a certain number of years, or until you are able to return to work.

Avoiding Pitfalls

Research before you act.
At this time, you should research what your company offers, and gain a clear picture of your benefits. Even if you think you understand them, ask questions. You'll need to design a solid strategy. Your financial survival will depend on whether you have a plan.

Clearly identify the stages of your illness.

For people who suffer with debilitating chronic illness, it's important to come to terms with the stages of its progression. You must be able to recognize when your body is beginning to decline. It must be faced head on. The natural desire to listen to false hope must be set aside. It will be up to you to understand how close you are to reaching the point at which you can no longer work.

Do not forecast your departure.
Don't share news of your illness or your impending departure in the workplace or anywhere else, except your therapist, doctor and family. Keep your health situation and plans for the future completely personal and private, as office gossip is taken directly to management and HR staff. Rumors tend to travel straight to the top of the organization; you'd be surprised how much the management knows about you. Before you know it, there might be planned layoffs. Your name could be on the next layoff list, because of something you've shared about your health status. Companies will often purge older employees and bring in new young workers, in an effort to reduce the number of employees who are likely to file health care and disability claims.

Don't confide in anyone at work.
We spend so much time at work that many workers view the work environment as a second home. Coworkers, especially those who are friendly and supportive, may begin to feel like your second family. However, when push comes to shove, a survival of the fittest mentality will kick in. Your coworkers may be in competition with you. They may envy your position or your salary. They are not your real family. Be careful. Watch what you say to your colleagues, even those you view as close friends. Placing too much trust in a coworker could cause you to lose your financial future.

Leave work while you are a full-time employee.
If you try to keep working beyond the point at which you are no longer able to work, you may be asked to leave work. This is the last thing you would want to happen. You can be demoted, transferred, or terminated on the grounds of poor performance. As soon as you feel too ill to perform your job, or when your illness is becoming visible to coworkers, you must go on disability leave. You must do this while you still hold a full-time position in order to keep full benefits that include medical, life, and long-term disability insurance.

Don't sign off on part-time hours or short-term disability.
At some point, you will have to tell your employer that you're ill. This is a crucial step in your career, and by making this step at the right time and in the right way, you can avoid falling into financial oblivion. Your employer might verbally assist you through your short-term disability paperwork. They may offer to help you lessen your workload. It's very likely they'll ask you to sign off on an easier schedule. Agreeing to this may be a serious mistake that you'll regret for the rest of your life.

Form a solid relationship with your doctor.
He or she will be an important teammate in your new life. A new destiny is about to unfold, full of lessons, trials, and triumphs. Your private doctor will become a best friend and their medical documentation will be used to verify and uphold your disability claim. You will need objective medical information, including laboratory results, MRI(s), Nuclear Medicine or Radiology test documentation or neurological assessments. And the key is an assessment of your activities of daily living.

Step by Step Guide to Exit Work

Step 1: Don't tell anyone at work about your impending departure until you have reached Step 6.

Step 2: Discuss your potential disability with your physician, who will become the protective partner for you the entire length of time you are unable to work. Be sure your physician agrees that you are disabled.

Step 3: Request a short-term leave, medical or disability request form(s) from management or HR.

Step 4: Fill out the patient's portion of the short-term leave or medical leave by having your physician fill out the company's disability form(s).

Step 5: Return the completed forms to management or HR. Do not negotiate.

Step 6: Prepare for your new life, in which the priorities are taking care of your health and managing all the documentation and financial issues of life on disability.

Conclusion

A decline in your health is leading you towards an inability to work. Leaving the workplace and filing a disability claim requires courage and consideration. Chronic injury and illness can be a roller-coaster. Don't rely on or confide in your coworkers or managers. Rely on your doctor to provide support and advice, while you make the decision and commit to it.

Once you know, in your heart and body, that your healthy working days are drawing to an end, it's time to execute a strategic and graceful exit. It's essential that you openly express your expectations, fears, needs, and practical and economic concerns to your spouse and other family members, as they will be greatly impacted by these changes.

Chapter 5
Mental Health

By now, you should be fully aware that your physical issues won't be the only concerns you will be facing. When you become disabled, you will find that a great mental and spiritual weight of confusion, anxiety, and stress has been dropped on your shoulders. Because you are undergoing what is surely considered a *major life event,* it is in your interest to find a coach, psychologist, or counselor, who can join with the others, who are playing critical supporting roles in your life's drama.

As with many of the things you'll need to deal with in one way or another when you are disabled, it won't be easy. You will likely need to shop around and try a few professionals, to see if they are helpful or in tune to your particular needs and requirements. Be wary of working with a therapist, for example, who only seems intent on giving you some sort of medication.

Once you do make a choice on who will be entrusted to your care, you should keep something else in mind. When you receive "therapy," "life coaching," or "counseling" from a trained individual, you should not simply be looking to take that person's advice without any real questions. Rather, you should see him or her as an individual, who can guide you through whatever issues you might have, as well as how you approach or interact with others.

When you get this kind of support, it is more akin to what an athletic coach or mentor has to offer, rather than somebody who is simply telling you what you should or should not be doing. This sort of assistance will help you identify relevant needs and issues, enabling you to zero in on the various things you can improve on, and decisions you might want to make for the benefit of your immediate needs, and the sake of your future.

Still, regardless of how much help you get from others, you will have to keep in mind that you will be in the midst of a major life incident that is wholly unfamiliar, and likely very traumatic. You will need to occasionally take time to step back, pause and reflect, or, perhaps, to put the brakes on any negative momentum.

If you feel things are becoming overwhelming, you should try to remain calm and listen to yourself. Allow your spirit and mind to rest and settle back from the highly charged atmosphere that a dramatic change in circumstances can sometimes, bring about. If that doesn't work, of course, then you should seek the assistance of a qualified professional.

You will be required to rely on friends, family, and you're your doctor, and counselor as primary human connections and supporters that you will need in order to engage and manifest the BEST and surpass the barriers that lie ahead. The storm is circling your mental and physical abilities and your dance movements must expand to include a trusted life coach or counselor.

In the next chapter, you will meet and follow Gloria Carter, whose chronic medical condition begins to worsen.

Chapter 6
Gloria Carter's First Week Homebound

Gloria Carter pushed her hair out of her face and took a deep breath of the misty morning air. The forty-eight-year-old San Franciscan had suffered all her life with congenital cerebral palsy. She had awakened early, sparked by a desire to get things done. She thought she might pay a few bills, even though she was still awaiting her disability payment from the insurance company.

As she eased herself up onto her elbows, a wave of dizziness swept over her. She fell back onto the pillows, a numbing chill rippling through her body. Her mind went blank, and she stared at the ceiling. Not a hint of dawn peeked through the bedroom blinds; the moon must still be hiding behind the clouds. The room was as dark as life on disability with advanced multiple sclerosis. She closed her eyes and took another deep breath. She had spent the last few days rearranging the home office she'd neglected during busier times, and this was probably why she felt so exhausted.

Gloria's glowing career as a software product manager flashed before her eyes. She had designed a software tool for creating and editing digital illustrations and written a marketing white paper that drew in hundreds of new clients. She had wept as she received the employee excellence award two years ago.

"You worked so hard for this bonus," a coworker had said.

"The hardest thing I ever accomplished," Gloria said, as her heart swelled.

"You deserve this."

"I haven't done too badly for someone with only two years of college. I'm so lucky."

"Luck has nothing to do with it. You're brilliant."

"I'm naïve about so many things." Gloria blushed. "I couldn't have done it without the help of the whole team."

Then, motor coordination issues had gradually seeped into her workdays. At first, the tiredness and her limp were barely noticeable. Months passed. Sometimes, she left the office an hour early. Another month went by. By now, she was leaving two hours early.

"Are you gaining weight?" Co-workers furrowed their brows and searched her face.

She shrugged. "I'm on a special diet."

That was over a year ago when it was still possible to evade their questions, before she gained forty pounds in three weeks. She began leaving the office halfway through each workday. That's when her perfect world had come crashing down. She could still feel the hollow disappointment in the pit of her stomach.

She prayed that the queasy feelings would subside. "Help me make it through this day," she whispered to her cat, who perched atop Gloria's chest as if listening to her heart. She scratched the top of Calico's head and, with a shaky hand, stroked the fur on her neck and back. "I'm so glad you're here for me. I don't know what's going to happen to me."

She glanced at the clock on her dresser. It was time to feed her beloved companion. Determined to get the day started, she raised herself up again. Calico vaulted to the floor and paced at the foot of the bed. Gloria eased her legs over the side of the bed. Her nerves tingled. Calico pranced back and forth, as the dim morning sun warmed the room.

"Are you hungry, honey?" She pushed aside the thought of the deadly neural condition eating away at her spinal column and gave her cat a loving look.

A few weeks before her 48th birthday, she had filed the requisite medical leave forms and resigned herself to the long wait for the state and long-term insurance disability to come through. That is if it ever came through at all.

The morning's silence was punctured by the chug-chug, roll-roll, ring-ring sounds of the trolley-car, pounding past her second-floor Victorian flat. Gloria loved the city's unique charm. She had especially loved riding the trolley to work every morning. The sounds revived and cheered her, and she felt her energy renewed. She planned to write about this new episode in her life. She loved to write. Expressing her emotions always released her feelings of fear and anger.

"We're going to get a few things done today," she declared to Calico, who responded with a squeaky purr.

Feeling strangely unrefreshed, even after 12 hours' sleep, Gloria forced her body upright. Teetering on her unstable legs, she moaned. The pitter-pat of Calico's paws followed. She felt around on the nightstand for the nine pills she had set out the night before. Clutching them in one hand, she leaned on the table for a moment, while she caught her breath. She slipped the pills into her pocket and stumbled to the kitchen.

"Here you go, sweet thing." She scooped cat food from the bag and dropped it into Calico's bowl. She bent down and patted her little head, wondering whether she'd get up at all if it wasn't for Calico. "Looks like you're almost out of food. I'll go to the store later."

She filled a glass with water and shuffled through the high-ceilinged flat. As she groggily entered the office, she was greeted by the sight of the papers piled up on the desk beside the dusty computer. She placed the glass on the desk and mustered her strength, wincing in pain as she eased herself into her brown leather chair. Recalling how she'd once loved coming into this room each morning, Gloria flipped the computer on. She scooped the pills from her pocket and slipped them into her mouth. She took the seven multicolored ones first, followed by the two white pills. Gloria gulped down the glass of water to wash away the bitter taste of the dissolving pills. She pinched her nose to stop herself from gagging at the taste. She typed a few pages of her story, pausing often to rest, leaning back in her chair.

David, her therapist, had counseled her during her high-tech career. These days, their weekly sessions focused on the stressful fallout of her decision to go on disability. As well as the stress of quitting her job and filing the necessary paperwork, she had undergone many lifestyle changes. Her life had revolved like clockwork around her work schedule, and the reward structure of her job gave her life meaning. She had also sold her car in order to reduce her cost of living. Without the cost of maintaining a car and paying for car insurance, her expected monthly disability pay would stretch to cover the cost of her keeping her home. Thus, her universe had shrunk considerably in more ways than one. David had suggested she begin to write about her experiences, as a way of dealing with her losses and the pain of adjustment.

A barrage of e-mails awaited Gloria. "Let's see." She sighed and opened a new window. She scanned the news and clicked on a link to donate to those affected by a recent hurricane. She donated 100.00 dollars before closing the window. That felt good. She still had some sick pay and vacation pay coming in from her old job, and she was glad she could help someone else in need.

She swiveled her desk chair around to face the window and drank in the view of her eccentric neighborhood. Her heartbeat quickened, as she gazed out across the San Francisco Bay. The sun edged the horizon with a tangerine tint, sketching shadows across the water. Alcatraz Island shimmered in the distance. She reveled in the picture-perfect view of the ocean, bits of fog, and the towering lighthouse beacon.

Looking off into the distance, she imagined she could see Marin, and Angel Island, as well as the neighboring kingdoms across the Bay.

She rotated back to her desk and adjusted her reading glasses. Her heart grew heavy. "Let's look at the bills." She rasped and coughed, growing lightheaded, as she strained to read the small print. She wished her bills weren't quite so high. Opening the desk drawer, she took out her checkbook and wrote out some checks.

Calico jumped into her lap. "Oh!" Gloria jumped. Rubbing Calico's ear, she stared into her cat's yellow eyes. "Yes, I haven't forgotten. I'll go to the store soon."

She opened more envelopes. "Oh my God! How could I miss the water payment?" She hastily wrote another check and tucked it into an envelope. She rested her head in her hands, which were shaking.

Calico jumped onto the desk and stretched out under the desk lamp.

"Mommy missed a bill last month." Gloria felt a tear squeeze from her eyes. "What would I do if I couldn't afford to keep you?" Her voice faltered, and a chill spread through her heart. She rubbed Calico's soft fur, feeling soothed by her pet's warmth.

Gloria opened the remaining letters, and her lips curled into a smile. "Some good news, Calico," she said. She glanced at the clock on the wall. It was almost eleven. Soon, it would be time for her nap.

The phone rang, making them both jump. Calico lifted her head and pricked up her ears. Gloria coughed and cleared her throat. The phone jangled again. "It's just the phone, Calico," Gloria said, lifting the receiver. "Hi, this is Gloria."

"Gloria? This is Deborah Wilson, I'm a qualified registered nurse."

Deborah's voice sounded pleasant. It reminded Gloria of her mother's voice soothing her during her childhood, providing solace after Gloria skinned her knee on the front steps. The mention of the word *nurse* made Gloria feel safe. A sense of security flooded her chest. This nurse was managing her case. Soon, she'd receive her first disability check in the mail. "I'm so glad you called," Gloria said.

"United Casualty Disability Insurance has assigned me as your case manager. I'll be processing your short to long-term disability claim."

Gloria frowned. "Processing my claim? Didn't I already qualify for disability? I already received a letter of confirmation in the mail. I don't understand. I thought receiving the letter meant I had filled out all of the forms correctly. Was some information missing?" She took out a sheet of paper and smoothed it out in front of her. She would write everything down so she didn't miss anything or make a mistake.

"The letter stated that your short term-leave was awarded. Now, I just need to review your file to determine whether you qualify for a long-term claim."

Gloria's heart skipped a beat, and her stomach twisted itself into a knot. "You mean I'm not on disability yet? I'm sorry, this is so confusing."

"I understand that this is all very complicated," Deborah said sweetly. "I'm here to help you. That's why I'm calling to introduce myself. Is this a good time for you?"

"Yes. Well, to be honest, I'm a bit tired and my head is spinning a little, but this is as good a time as any." She felt a tinge of discomfort. Had she already made a mistake? She decided to let Deborah take the lead. That would be the best way to gain her approval. "I'd like to be as helpful as I can."

"That's lovely, Gloria. I just have a few quick questions."

"I'm ready," Gloria said, eager to reach a swift resolution.

"How are you feeling today?" Deborah asked.

"I'm doing fine." Gloria slipped into her old habit of feigning an upbeat manner. Even though her words had a hollow ring, she'd learned that people are expected to exchange morning pleasantries, so they could move on with their day.

"Okay, then. You're feeling fine?"

Gloria could hear the rustle of papers. She could feel her energy fading with every passing moment. She needed to rest, but she wasn't sure if saying this to Deborah would help or hurt her case.

"You sound a little hoarse," Deborah said, sounding concerned. "Have you been up long?"

"I've been up for a few hours. I have coughing spells in the morning."

"What color is your sputum?"

"It's clear or whitish. My doctor did some tests for infections, but these came back negative." Since Deborah was a nurse, perhaps she could shed some light on this. "What do you think?"

"Your physician is Dr. Greene. Is that correct?"

"Yes." Gloria frowned, surprised at Deborah's sudden change of tack. "Your records show that you've recently gained a considerable amount of weight."

"Yes." Gloria coughed so hard that it made her gag. She covered the mouthpiece.

"What is your current weight?"

"You just said you've seen it in my records. Why do you need to ask me?"

"It's just for verification purposes. How long have you been ill?"

"Why are you asking me all these questions? I wrote everything on the form." Getting mad at Deborah probably wasn't helping her case. She took a deep breath and tried to speak calmly. "I've been getting sicker and sicker for over a year now. Everything makes me feel tired."

"I see." Deborah's voice was deathly calm. "I'm sorry to hear that," she added. The sweetness of her voice now seemed menacing, rather than comforting. "Well, I think that's enough for now. I don't want to tire you out. I have enough here to initiate processing your case. I'll check in with you again in a few weeks. In the meantime, feel free to call me if you have any questions."

Gloria's stomach felt like a stone. "A few weeks? What do you mean you're just starting?"

"As I explained, we are beginning to process your long-term claim."

"But I don't have a few weeks. I really need the money. I'm behind in paying bills, and I need to hire someone to help me around the house."

"I fully understand. We'll talk soon. Have a wonderful day."

Gloria put down the phone. Her shoulders slumped forward. She crumpled the blank sheet of paper and tossed it into the trash can. **What had just happened? What had she done?**

In her next session with David, she let her fears show. Her eyes had dark circles underneath them.

"How are you, Gloria?"

"I finally talked with my case manager."

"How did it go?"

"Horrible, I think. I have a really bad feeling about her. I told her I was feeling fine! It was a knee-jerk reaction. I'm just so used to always pretending that I'm fine." She closed her eyes and shook her head.

"I'm sure it was fine. You'll hear back from her soon. Meanwhile, why don't you write it out and release some pressure?"

"You read my mind! I've been making notes."

David smiled. "You might create a bestseller."

"A horror story," Gloria quipped. "I'll get some rest and start writing it tomorrow."

"The important thing is that you have a plan. Our time's up. We'll continue this next week."

Gloria felt calmer after the session. That evening, she retired to her bedroom and relaxed in front of the TV. Every commercial sold a product aimed at people on the go, whether at work or play. She felt more aware than ever, of her life's new emptiness, her isolation from the rest of the world.

Chapter 7
Your Physical Health

Before a discourse about qualifying for disability and living on disability, it is important to spell out the need to pay attention to your health issues. While you have the time, you can work on those things you've ignored. Take a daily walk and try to eat better and get to a healthy weight. From an evolutionary point of view, humans are gifted machines, bestowed with attributes and abilities that can help you move mountains. We possess the physical structure and dexterity to accomplish tasks that, at first glance, seem undoable. Not all of us have superior musculature, of course. But regardless of whether we are naturally blessed with muscles or not, we owe it to ourselves to nurture and enhance our physical being and to maintain it as meticulously as we would a finely-tuned engine. When you exercise physically, it maintains your mental health and energy.

Even with an injury or illness, we should care for the human apparatus, just as we would a rare Ferrari, cleaning and tuning ourselves up at least three times a week.

As President John F. Kennedy noted, *"Physical fitness is not only one of the most important keys to a healthy body, it is the basis of dynamic and creative intellectual activity."*

Maintain a healthy body. It's important to walk, stretch, body build and work out, in order to realize our future potential.

Modify Your Physical Habits

Examine the things you do habitually; alcohol use, dental cleaning, and physical exercise. No matter the habit you wish to modify, using this template of alcohol use can be applied.

For those who realize that substance use must change, the first step is figuring out what we would like to limit or stop. After all, we are the governors over everything in our lives. But it is only after we make the decision that things can happen. Use your character tools of intention, strength, and determination. That doesn't mean it will be easy. Anyone who is or has ever been hooked on a substance like alcohol or dangerous or reckless drug use knows how difficult it can be to end the addiction habit. It can help to know the right strategies or have access to the right kind of help.

One approach could be called the *substitution method*. Let's say you frequently use or are addicted to alcohol. When you get the urge to drink, try replacing some or all of the relevant enhancers with a healthier alternative. If, for example, it's Friday night when you normally consume an excessive number of cocktails, try replacing the third drink with clear, fresh water or juice. If you repeat this process each time, soon, you will have established a routine that makes you feel better, and which you can feel good about. The positive reinforcement is that you've accomplished a small goal in reduction (and probably saved some money too). Mastery comes with practice.

Sometimes, of course, we can't do it ourselves. Indeed, contrary to what you are often led to believe, we should never fear to ask for help. That means reaching out and getting assistance from friends and family, health professionals, or those who have aided other habitual drinkers in their efforts to get clean. In many cases, a mentor or life coach can help you understand who you are and what you need, then walk you through the darkest places in your mind to find the light.

Chapter 8
Gloria's 11th Week Homebound

Gloria Carter's nerves were thoroughly shot. Another month had passed, and her disability payment was still nowhere to be seen. Each morning, she opened her mailbox with trembling hands. The bills were piling up. She was struggling to keep up with the household chores. She needed to hire someone to help her out, but where would the money come from? What if she fell so far behind on her rent that she got evicted? She was sick and weak. How would she relocate to another apartment? Unanswered questions haunted her. Every day, she documented her story.

The rattling of the bay windows woke her. One story below, a street trolley thundered past. Early commuters shuttled through quaint San Francisco neighborhoods toward the bustling financial center downtown. She loved the trolley sounds and looked forward each morning to being embraced by their San Francisco charm.

The Social Security disability check was due to arrive on the third of each month. Today was the fifteenth. Still nothing. Standing in front of her mailbox, Gloria rifled through a stack of bills. Her stomach turned, and her hands shook. This couldn't be happening.

Had they stopped her disability pay? Perhaps, the check had gotten lost in the post.

The phone rang. The sound made her panic, and she was briefly overwhelmed by a coughing fit. She waited for it to subside and cleared her throat before picking up the receiver. "Gloria Carter speaking."

"Good morning, Gloria. This is Deborah Wilson from UCD." Deborah's voice sounded like a recording.

"Hi, Deborah. I'm so glad you called. I've been waiting for a long time to hear from you." Gloria covered the phone and cleared her throat. Her patience had paid off. Here was the good news at last.

"Just as I promised, I'm getting back to you on your disability claim. You're sounding very energetic."

A chill spread through her body. "Oh, sure," she said. "I try my best over the phone. I have these miracle medications, and they give me a bit of extra kick, especially in the mornings."

"You sound just great this morning," Deborah said.

"Thank you," Gloria said, though Deborah's tone had sounded almost accusatory. She felt a sharp pang of anxiety. Had she done something wrong?

"That's really what I wanted to speak to you about. It seems to us you may have exaggerated the seriousness of your condition. For a start, you claimed to have gained a significant amount of weight—"

"No, *you* were the one who said that!" Gloria felt like her head was about to explode. "You said—"

"Your weight has only increased by 15 %," Deborah said sternly.

"Oh?" Gloria wondered if this was good or bad.

"Your lab results indicate that your condition is fair," Deborah said sourly. Gloria pictured a woman with a puckered mouth, sitting stiffly at her desk, her hair scraped back into a bun. "Everything's still within the normal range."

Gloria's heart began to race. "Oh. That's strange, because—I mean, you've seen the results from my blood work!"

"You said you were feeling great the last time I called."

Flashing back to that phone call, Gloria realized how she must have sounded. She shouldn't have told Deborah she felt okay. Snippets of that conversation swirled in Gloria's mind. Out of courtesy, she had withheld the specifics of her illness, assuming all her medical problems were documented in the doctor's records.

"You sound fit and strong," hissed Deborah.

"I am. I mean, I was just making everyday water cooler conversation, the way I'm used to." Gloria stumbled over her own words. How could she save herself?

"You said you wanted to try to work a little. Perhaps, an hour or so a day."

It hit her in the gut. "How can you think I'm well enough to work?" Gloria sensed she was digging the hole even deeper. *I have to correct this thing right now*, she thought. "I was being polite! I'm sick, but I'm used to hiding it."

"Um, so why did you tell me you were able to work intermittently?" Deborah asked.

"Are you crazy? I can't be on any kind of schedule." Panic swirled in her stomach and for a moment she felt like she was going to throw up. "There's no predictability in my day." Her fear intensified.

"That sounds like a time management issue or a lack of motivation. Neither of those things constitutes a health condition. We want to help you, but we can't unless we can determine what exactly is wrong with you," Deborah said.

Gloria felt like crying. "That's just the thing! I don't know what's wrong with me. I have cerebral palsy," her voice trembled.

"Well, are you or are you not able to work on some days?" Deborah insisted.

Gloria was beginning to hate this woman. "How can you ask me that?" Waves of emotion rose from the pit of her stomach. "No! I can't work some of the time. My life is impossible right now. I'm so sick, but I don't know what's wrong with me."

"We don't know either." Deborah's voice echoed in the earpiece.

"I suffer every day!" Gloria's voice rose. "Almost every single moment of every single day." Her heart was pounding in her chest.

"We can't read your mind. All we can do is look at your results and your records."

Gloria's palms were sweating. She wondered what exactly was documented in her chart and in the insurer's records. Did they just cherry-pick what they wanted to see? The short-term disability checks were inconsequential, and her savings were running out fast. Would she end up living in shelters and begging for food? She was already so sick; how could she live on the edge of survival? "It's on record, though. I have cerebral palsy."

"A lot of people have that and can still work."

"I understand that, but it's different for different people. Believe me, I would rather be working. I would rather not be sick." Gloria tightened her grip on the receiver.

"We want to believe you," Deborah said quietly, "but we have no reason to. You're making this very hard on yourself."

Gloria keeled over as if she had been stabbed in the stomach. Those last words echoed in her head. She ended the call. It was over. She could feel her energy draining out of every pore. A sinking feeling came over her. Had another horror story just unfolded? Had they dropped her?

She did a quick search and found a lawyer who specialized in disability insurance claims.

Chapter 9
Should I Get a Lawyer?

If you have any sort of encounter with the justice system, one question you must always consider is whether you need legal representation. You will not want to find yourself with the short end of the stick because you didn't have someone by your side who understands everything that is going on and who can ensure you don't do anything that might put you needlessly at risk.

But that is not the only time you should be making this assessment. You should also ask the question before moving forward with a disability claim. As when dealing with the police or the courts, if you make a misstep or otherwise say the wrong thing, however innocently, it can leave you on the defensive and make it difficult, if not impossible, to get justice.

With this in mind, below are three reasons why you should be saying "yes" to having a knowledgeable advocate on your side:

Reason 1: You are making it clear you are not playing games.

As Gloria Carter learned – the hard way – it's important to get legal representation early on so that your disability insurer knows you are serious and ready to do battle with them for whatever you are owed.

Once a lawyer agrees to take on your case, you will need to pay your legal representative a retainer, which represents an upfront advance against potential legal fees and expenses you might owe as a result of his efforts on your behalf.

While this may well be challenging, to say the least, especially with all of the medical and other expenses you may suddenly be faced with, it nonetheless makes a great deal of sense to arrange it, even if it means borrowing to cover the cost.

Why?

Because once your provider is notified that you have secured a member of the legal profession to represent you, your filed claim will immediately be **flagged** at their end. From that moment on, the insurance company's employees will be aware that they need to direct all communications regarding your case to your attorney and comply with requests as required, or else face the risk that they themselves, may be subjected to costly legal actions.

Playing on claimant fears and non-responsiveness

For those who don't have a professional by their side, the insurance company may take the view that there is little to be gained by playing fair. Most likely, they will take a harder line with respect to claims where there is no lawyer involved and will go so far as to reject most of them, at least initially.

In fact, insurers have found that many claimants simply do not respond to initial denials, or they decide to abandon their claims after just one official-sounding and a legalese-filled letter from the insurer. Because this has proved to be a great way for them to reduce payouts and, thus, to boost profits, they have come up with a range of ingeniously cold-hearted communications to prospective claimants that would make most people's hearts stop. Below is one example of the kind of correspondence you might receive after submitting a claim for benefits:

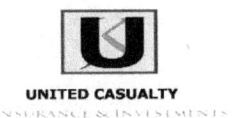

UNITED CASUALTY
INSURANCE & INVESTMENTS

☎ 1 5 9   856
✉ info@jacksonkennedy.com
🌐 www.jacksonkennedy.com
📍 P.O. Box 3˙ 3, hill street, NY

Claimant: Gregory Madison	Date:	12/20/2012
Case #: 900122	SS #:	XXX-XX-2908
Claim #: 000771	Employer:	City Builders

Dear Mr. Gregory Madison,

We have reviewed your claim # 00771 for short-term disability benefits and have not found adequate medical evidence or clinical lab values necessary to authorize your claim.

Therefore, your claim has been closed as of the date of this notification letter.

Sincerely,

Dr. Jerry Carlson
Medical Claims Examiner
United Casualty Insurance

It isn't just the communications they send out that are designed to make you call it quits. Below, is some real-life feedback regarding the actions – and non-actions – that insurers have taken through the years in an effort to prevent prospective claimants from getting paid in accordance with the terms of the policies they hold:

- "All I keep getting is the runaround. Calls and letters are not returned. No one is trying to help me at all."

- "I believe my disability insurer follows the 'let's deny everything' approach. If they happen to call, their standard operating procedure is to place you on hold and then disconnect the call. If they manage to stay on the line, they make ridiculous statements such as "we can't process your claim" or "your claim is being denied because no treating doctor is specified."

- "I've been out of work for two months due to maternity leave. The insurance company has been saying for some time now that my medical records haven't been faxed over to them. I called them last week and the person who answered the phone said they had my records and were looking them over. Today, they said, once again, that they don't have my documents and, as a result, my case is denied."

- "Dealing with the disability insurance company has been the worst experience of my life. It's probably going to cause me to file for bankruptcy even though the facts of my case are pretty clear.

    First, I fainted and got a concussion. After that, I lost consciousness and somebody called 911. I've been to two emergency rooms since then and have been told to stay home from work until I get clearance. My neurologist would not clear me, however, and I was eventually referred to a neuro-psychotherapist.
    Finally, after being off work for more than 10 weeks, I was allowed to return to my job. Meanwhile, my insurer is doing everything they can not to pay me. They are seeking all kinds of information about me that has nothing to do with my head injury.

- "I have paid into disability insurance for 11 years. I am now filing a claim for the first time, and it has become the worst nightmare ever. Aside from the fact that my assigned claim manager never calls me back, despite promising to do so, I have been fighting to get this taken care of for almost a month, even though they have all of the documentation on file that they requested."

- "I recently filed for benefits. My claim was denied because the insurer has a 180-day window during which I had to file. This requirement was not in place when I purchased my policy."

- "At first, they sat on my claim, with one delay or another since May, even though my VA primary care doctor verified, in writing, the details of my injuries and the days I was out of out of work during that time." Eventually, they simply denied it."

- "I was placed on medical leave last September. I kept hearing from the insurer that my 'records were not received.'" After six months, I was finally able to get this sorted out. Not long after that, they denied my claim."

- "My disability insurer needs to be investigated and hit with a class action lawsuit for, among other things, deliberately denying valid claims. Their favorite excuse is that they haven't received anything from the doctor. This is quite alarming. How is it that so many people's documents have not been received despite the doctor's offices having received confirmation that the faxes were transmitted successfully?"

- "Well, I had no problems getting paid out on my short-term insurance policy, which was covered by my employer. However, when it came to my long-term policy, which I purchased directly through the insurer, lots of games began as soon as the claims process started."

A word of warning: first and foremost, make sure you record everything you say on the phone and tell them you want written transcripts of any conversations you have with them.

Reason 2: You are handling the headaches to somebody else.

Rather than compound your misfortune, let your expert take the lead on the claim process, and put at least, some of the pressure back onto your insurer.

Reason 3: You are helping ensure it is a fair fight.

When your disability insurer gives you the runaround, it isn't just making it more difficult for you to collect what is rightfully yours. The many obstacles the company places in front of you, the redundant and ridiculous requests, and the way your claim is bundled and addressed, creates considerable stress that can be almost overwhelming when you are struggling with health issues.

As in a wide range of legal matters, it is important to have somebody on your side who knows how the game is supposed to be played, and what you should say or do when pressing a claim for disability benefits. When, and if the insurer sends an inspector to your home to verify what you say about the things you can't do, you will be much better off if you have an expert by your side, who can help you navigate and control the conversation. In addition, your representative is likely to be adept at ensuring that all the necessary follow-ups and documentation requests are handled properly.

The Downside of Legal Representation

Admittedly, there are times when having an expert on your side will leave you with little more than another bill to pay. For one thing, you could be lucky enough – in a manner of speaking – to have a support organization nearby that provides legal and other assistance to individuals with issues like yours at little or little cost.
But assuming that is not the case, the odds of prevailing when making a claim will likely increase if you hire a professional advocate, who understands how the process is supposed to work. To be sure, this kind of expertise doesn't come cheap, nor does it guarantee you will prevail. In fact, you could end up in more difficult financial straits than you were in when you started the process.

The fact is, however, that it is difficult to do it on your own, and there are plenty of risks along the way. While you can't hand everything off to the lawyer once he is engaged – you will still need to fill out forms and provide other information and documentation – he will likely be in the best position to ensure everything is handled properly. Under the circumstances, making this investment would seem to be quite beneficial, especially when you start receiving regular monthly payments for a potentially long time to come.

Conclusion

Let's face it, most of us have probably had to deal with all sorts of cloudbursts and stormy maelstroms in our lives. More than likely, we have pulled back our shoulders, raised our chins high, and linked hands to work through it with one expert, or another at our sides. There is no reason why the disability claim process can't be yet, one more way for you – or any of us – to do the same.

In order to break through the cloudburst, you must reach out one more time and find the best and most trustworthy legal resource possible. Link arms and intentionally build the protective barriers that will produce eventual justice.

Chapter 10
Insurance Company Paranoia

Gloria Carter felt the twinges of confusion and paranoia in her gut, and was on high alert, even though she had Jeff Atkinson, Esq., at her side. More than likely, you will experience something just like it, particularly during interactions with your insurance company and, perhaps, your employer.

It is perfectly understandable why you might feel this way. History suggests that insurers try to shake prospective claimants out of the system, anyway they can because that helps to boost their bottom lines. They also go to great lengths to avoid paying out funds, even if it is clear to everyone involved that this practice is wrong.

Sadly, more than half of all filed disability claims are not completed or honored because of all the hoops, obstacles, and confusion claimants must suffer through to receive their contracted benefits. Those who were making good money – say, a six-figure annual salary – before they became disabled are generally targeted for intense scrutiny. To heighten the odds that the insurance company won't get away with it in your case, you'll want to consider the following:

1. **Bond with your doctor.** They are the gatekeeper who wields the medical science that will justify your claim and help get it approved.

2. **Get a lawyer.** More often than not, it does not make sense to do it alone. Find a local lawyer who specializes in your type of disability claims.

3. **Take notes and plan efficiently.** Your job is now the disability claim process and you must be diligent about documenting the calls you have made and the letters you receive. You should also maintain an up-to-date list of actions and communications you need to take care of or have already completed. By keeping it near you or at your desk, it will serve as a regular reminder of what you must do to keep your claim alive.

4. **Prepare for any phone calls you will receive.** Employers and insurers like to call claimants who are ill or incapacitated. When you're sick or in pain, phone conversations can be confusing or hard to remember, and your misunderstanding about technical instructions given orally over the phone could be used as a reason to drop your claim.

    Even innocent words can come back to haunt you if you are not careful about what you say. If you respond to the friendly question, "How are you?" with the innocent retort "I'm fine, thank you," an insurer may well document your response and use it against you in future.

5. **Prepare for whatever correspondence you will receive**. Employers and insurance companies are known for sending letters, requesting information that has tight deadlines. Worse still, the letters are often peppered with the sort of legalese that may send a ripple of emotional turmoil through you. While it is easy to become frightened and frustrated, take a step back and weigh your options, including talking to your lawyer, before responding.

6. **Get your forms in order.** You and your doctor will be required to fill out various documents, including any number of forms where the same

questions are asked repeatedly. If you leave fields blank or do not get certain forms back from your physician in a timely manner, your insurer will likely try to close your claim and leave you wanting.

7. **Be prepared for video surveillance.** Insurance companies will often hire local videographers to spend time outside your home, recording your activities. They will be assessing how healthy you look, including whether you are walking without assistance and lifting objects. If they find you engaging in running, sports, or exercise, they will assume you've lied on your claim for benefits and will likely reject it.

8. **Be prepared for a potential neighbor, friend and family surveillance.** Insurers have been known to befriend those who are closest to you and ask probing or personal questions that could lead, even innocently, to a denial of your claim.

9. **Get to know the terminology.** The disability insurance world is rife with technical terms, legalese, and industry jargon that could easily confuse anyone who does not have the requisite knowledge or training of a lawyer or insurance professional. If you don't know what something means, don't be afraid to ask or otherwise, look it up.

10. **Ensure your bank and credit card transactions are consistent with your claim.** The insurance company will likely review your financial transactions to see what you are spending your money on. If you are regularly traveling or going to the gym and your disability claim states that you are homebound, there's a good chance these expenditures will be used against you.

11. **Document everything.** Disability claims are a legal matter and you should receive specific instructions and requests from both the employer and insurer. Having the documentation on hand will help you clearly understand what they are looking for. If they tell you something over the phone or in a meeting, ask for a letter or fax spelling out what they want. Once you have this in writing, you have some protection, enhancing your prospects for succeeding with the claim.

Chapter 11
Get Your House in Order

It is time to get your house in order, Canadian clinical psychologist, Dr. Jordan Peterson, has said, and be prepared for any possibility during a time of uncertainty. His perspective certainly holds true when you are incapacitated, spending most of your time at home, and seriously working on your disability claim.

Your environs – from your home overall, to the room where you spend much of your time to the place where you store notes or write letters – should be your fortress, nurturing your energy and soul. Because you will have some good days and some very bad days, you must be able to refuel your courage and strengthen your character. Moreover, since you will be transforming your old life into one with new goals and aspirations, you'll want to rearrange your space to support the life-rebuilding process.

In this phase of your existence, there are things you can do to help regain at least some of the control that was taken away from you. Some are quite simple, but they can nonetheless make your new day job easier and decidedly less stressful. It is doubtful whether any of these ideas will catapult you into a luxurious manner of living, but they can make it easier to come to grips with a seemingly unmanageable situation. Having more control can give you a renewed self-esteem.

Desk or Work area

You should begin by assessing your surroundings, especially those areas where you will be spending a great deal of your time.

Where will you be making most of your calls, reading messages, and completing forms? For some, this might mean the bedroom. For others, it will be the kitchen table or home office. Regardless, you'll want to ensure you also keep your disability book, log or a diary app on your smart phone.

You'll also want to have a specific location for correspondence and files. In your new job, you will be required to manage a variety of needs, documents, and appointments. To ensure you can access them and refer to them as necessary, they can – or should – be organized by type or category (e.g., work-related letters, disability forms, life insurance forms, social security documents) and kept in folders or, for instance, accordion-sectioned paper-holders.

Records and Notes

It is also important that you maintain a file, organized chronologically, of any documentation and correspondence related to your claim, including your initial application; information from your employer; physician's statements; medical information that you submitted; letters from you, your insurer, and your attorney; and any supplemental forms you need to complete.

You should review this material often to catch and clarify details you might otherwise have missed and to note patterns of delays or denials. Keep in mind that you are legally entitled to have copies of everything your insurer has about you in their files, including internal memos, independent medical examination reports, and surveillance videos they might have obtained from private investigators. If you are denied access to any of this information, follow up with an attorney or your State insurance commissioner.

Disability Claim Log

One of the best ways to stay on top of things is to have a dedicated log. Take some time and find a nice folder or book that is the right size for you and handy to work with. Once it is ready, you should strive to document each and every call and action made or taken regarding your disability and the work you are no longer able to perform, including such items as post-employment COBRA medical benefits.

This process should be an essential part of your new life. Aside from logging conversations and calls, you will also want to make a record of every meeting you have and letter you send or receive to anyone involved in the process. Technology is your friend, and phone apps are useful. This may include state and federal disability agencies, short and long-term disability insurance providers, human resources personnel, life insurance companies, and any other parties that might be relevant to your case.

Although the primary goal of maintaining such a log is to help you stay on top of things, it will also serve as essential support for a process that may take months or even years to play out. By identifying what you have done and who you have interacted with, you can keep everyone, including the insurance provider, fully accountable. If or when a dispute occurs, you will have documentation at your fingertips that backs up your position.

Needless to say, if you don't have an organized system in place, you may forget certain key details, or lose track of your claims or the overall benefit process, especially if your disability turns out to be a major drain on your time, energy and life. Without this support mechanism in place, you could easily end up losing the benefits you deserve – and are entitled to.

Phone Numbers, Links and Addresses

It isn't just the content and nature of your interactions with others that matters, however. You're going to be contacting and calling numerous individuals, departments and organizations, most of which are likely new to you. These might include HR departments, benefits counselors, insurance agencies and doctors' offices.

In many cases, they may want forms and other documents sent to a range of different mailing addresses, including post office boxes, rather than to main office addresses. They may also want you to call certain phone numbers, depending on circumstances.

More often than not, many of these phone numbers, extensions, and addresses are difficult to find or are otherwise hidden. They do not necessarily jump out at you when you're reading thorough correspondence.

While you may feel like a detective when asking for a person's name and extension when speaking on the phone, it is important to get this information, especially if you are speaking with employees located deep in the recesses of larger organizations.

Reminders

If your mind is not working 100% or you have a great many things on your plate, you may find it makes sense to have reminders that tell you what has to be done each day. You may have pressing deadlines or need to take certain actions that really can't wait, such as mailing important letters, paying bills, making medical or other appointments, and taking medications.

Your health may also come into it: if you find your energy ebbs through the day, to the point where you can't even get out of bed when the afternoon is over, you'll likely want to sort out any number of things early on. Because chronic illness can affect each of us differently, you may find, for instance, that you're at your best around midday, or any other time in-between. Regardless, you'll want to plan things so you can make the most of your unique circumstances.

There are various ways you can stay on track. Perhaps you can get a small daily calendar or notebook. At night and at other times, place it next to your bed or some other place that you will always remember to look at, and have a dark pen nearby. Take time to record all the tasks that need to be done on any given day and then when you wake up, make sure you have a look.

Alternatively, you may want to get a little chalkboard and place it near your work area or buy some Post-it notepads, which you can leave, together with a pen, near your bed or where your phone is located. Each time you jot down something you need to do or remember, stick the reminder notes in your work area so you'll be sure to see them when the next day begins.

Nurturing Place

It is true that managing your disability claim is going to be your new job. But that doesn't necessarily mean you will be working every hour of the day. If you are like many of those who are disabled or seriously ill, you will likely be spending considerable time just being sick. If so, you may simply want to lie in bed or rest on a couch. Think about making this spot a comfortable haven that can help you to recover or simply get by.

Pillows, Blankets and Other Things

Even if you are spending the bulk of your time in bed, that doesn't necessarily mean you will be asleep or lying still. To ensure you can adapt to your daily needs and how you feel, secure plenty of pillows so you can prop yourself up in different positions. You may also want to get a small electric blanket for dealing with peripheral neuropathy or a fever, for when the days grow chilly. With the click of a button, you will experience soothing warmth – and psychological comfort.

Moreover, since this may end up as your home within a home, so to speak, you'll want to ensure you have shelves, TV trays, other resting places, and even a miniature refrigerator nearby. This will allow you to have a phone, pen, books, and a notepad handy, as well as access to medicines. With a set-up like this, you will be able to read mail and deal with bills and other paperwork while you're in bed, helping to ensure that important business won't somehow get missed.

Television

Let's face it: you're potentially going to be spending a lot of time on your own and/or dealing with your health. Under the circumstances, having access to digital cable television – along with a remote – may prove rather beneficial. If you are ill at night and can't sleep, you can turn the TV on, and flip through hundreds of channels, searching for content that may help you cope. Some shows will make you laugh – aiding your health – while others may simply capture your attention, taking your mind off your own circumstances.

Reading and Papers

It goes without saying that you'll have plenty to read through when you are dealing with your disability claim. Over time, you will likely receive letters, reports, and forms – many written in legalese and requiring considerable concentration – that you'll need to digest and follow up on. Aside from that, you may simply want to read for enjoyment. Either way, your bedroom setup should make it easy for you to go through what you can and pick things up later, if necessary.

The Fixings

You'll likely be spending plenty of time on your own, but that doesn't mean things will always be that way. Perhaps you will have professionals coming by to attend to your health, or friendly faces dropping in to see how you're doing.

Under the circumstances, you might want to have a chair or some other seating nearby. Of course, you don't have to wait for someone to show up: you can simply invite family and friends over to join you and to enjoy spending time together or simply to watch TV.

For your benefit and for theirs, however, you may also want to have a wastebasket on hand. Together with all of your own paper and other leftovers, having additional traffic coming through your room simply means there will be more stuff to throw away.

Medical Supplies

It will likely, vary depending on your particular condition, of course, but you will likely have to take certain medications on a daily or otherwise regular basis, and may also need to have other supplies, including those for infusions or IV drips, somewhere in the vicinity.

You probably won't want to have everything piled up high next to your bed, but you'll want to organize and store things in a place where they can readily be reached. You should have an easy way to reorder new supplies when you're running low.

Make Life Easy

For the most part, the key is to transform what could be a very challenging and labor-intensive mission into something that you are better able to handle. When you were healthy, you could have pushed yourself to get a lot more done each day. You might have filled your life with activities and other things successful people do to show others that they've made it. But now, you need to slow things down. It's time to get matters under control and make your new life easier – for you.

Chapter 12
The Morning Mail

Gloria Carter heard the familiar shuffle and flap of letters being pushed through the mail slot. *It's early today,* she thought as she slowly made her way down the stairs. White and yellow envelopes sprouted from the opening like a bouquet of flowers. She hoped they did not contain more bills, as her checking account contained only one hundred dollars.

She turned and began the slow climb to the top of the stairs. When she reached the top, she paused to flip through the stack, checking each return address. Yet another credit card offers, another bill, and—her stomach turned at the sight of the United Casualty Insurance logo and address. Weeks had passed since she had last heard from Jeff Atkinson. She stared at the letter.

What might this be? Is this going to ruin my day?

She weighed the envelope in her hand. It seemed larger and thicker than usual. Which kind of letter would be thicker, an acceptance or a denial? Her hands shook with fear and rage as she pried open the envelope and pulled out the contents. She smoothed out the pages, bracing herself to receive bad news.

Her heart began to sink as her eyes moved slowly down the page. A perforated line separated the white top two-thirds from the bluish bottom one-third. She blinked. Was she seeing what she thought she was seeing? She was! The check was made out for over twenty thousand dollars. It almost didn't seem real. *This can't be happening. It must be a mistake.*

She skimmed the letter.

"Dear Ms. Carter, we are pleased . . . your disability award . . . your first payment, including back pay due. . ."

This was it. Her very first long-term disability check!

She stood staring at it in disbelief for a few moments before going to the phone. She made a call to Jeff Atkinson's office. As she waited for him to pick up, she sat on the chair in the hallway. Was this really happening? Would she get paid every month from now on? She read and reread the letter, trying to find the catch.

"Good morning. Jeff Atkinson here."

"Jeff! My first check came in!"

"That's great," Jeff said. "You must be very relieved. Finally, after all that worry and waiting. Good luck with everything."

"Thank you! Goodbye."

She hung up the phone and stared at the wall opposite, still waiting for it to sink in. This was the best thing that had happened to her in so many months. She felt as if she had been struck by a benevolent bolt of lightning. It was like a dream. She had given up daring to even hope for a positive outcome, and now, all of a sudden, things had fallen into place. She felt the hellish uncertainty and torture of the past months fade away into a distant memory. She was bursting with happiness.

A few days later, Gloria walked into David's office with a bounce in her step and a grin on her face.

"You seem extremely chipper," David commented. "What's up?"

"I received my claim money! Including the back pay!"

"That's amazing. You must be so relieved. You've been through an awful lot. But you were patient, and it paid off. I'm excited for you!"

"Thank you so much for helping me to get through it. I couldn't have done it without you. I especially appreciate your suggestion to write everything down. That's what kept me sane. It helped me to process my emotions and to cope with all the stress."

"So now that this has been resolved, do you know what you want to do next?"

"Well, now that this part of my journey is finished, I'd like to develop my journal into a manuscript. I'll publish it as an e-book. The title will be *Get your Money!*"

David laughed. "Catchy, and to the point. Will you publish it under your real name or a pen name?"

"I'm allowed to earn royalties while on disability, but I might use an alias to protect my identity. I was thinking it might sell better under a man's name. I like the sound of Marla Parks."

David nodded approvingly. "Sounds personable, yet authoritative. You have this all worked out. Nothing can stop you now."

Gloria beamed at him. "It sure feels that way. I may treat myself to a glass of sherry tonight!"

Chapter 13
The Moment of Truth

Once your disability claim has been approved and is in process, the matter doesn't simply end there. For one thing, you must continue to prove you are disabled for as long as you are receiving payments, which means periodic follow-up visits to your doctor and related contacts with your insurer. Generally speaking, you must supply fresh medical evidence backing your claim every quarter or so. In addition, you will need to keep the insurer apprised of other matters, including income that comes your way.

When you get your award

Nevertheless, the fact is that you have finally gotten to the moment of truth and the result you have worked so hard to achieve. Typically, your first award notice will be mailed to you and will include a check covering what you are owed up to that point, including any payments due for the time during which you have been waiting or for the period of back pay that was covered, which can amount to months of payments.

Needless to say, it will be a happy day when the confirmation letter and the insurer's check arrives. Not long after, you will probably receive notice that your claim has been transferred to a disability benefits administrator at the insurance company, who will oversee the process of making sure you get your monthly benefit. For the time being, at least, the claim screening process and your efforts to prove your eligibility are over.

Automatic Deposits

Once your monthly benefits start coming in, you can ask the administrator to arrange for the payments to be automatically deposited in your bank. While it might seem reassuring to have a check in your hands, it makes sense to have it processed electronically to avoid delays or the prospect of it getting lost. It's worth remembering, for instance, what happened during the Anthrax scare of 2001, when many postal facilities were closed for days and letters were left to sit. How many disability checks went undelivered back then?

The process for arranging direct deposit tends to be relatively straightforward, requiring that you send a fax – or, in some cases, an email – detailing the specifics of your request. Presumably, you will have followed the plan in effect since the beginning of the disability claim process and recorded the numbers and email addresses you need to contact in your own records.

Overall, processing your request can take a month or two and typically involves you being sent a form that asks for information about your account, including the bank's "routing number" and the account number (if you don't have this information, a quick call to your bank can help you get it sorted out). Assuming there are no hiccups, once you sign and return the completed form to the insurer, you will soon begin receiving your funds electronically each month.

No Income

As a condition of your continued payments, you will have little choice but to report any income you receive to your disability administrator.

If you earn it through some kind of work, they will assert that you have breached the contract. Some claimants might feel they can get away with getting paid under the table, but if you are caught, you could lose your entire benefit, which is definitely not something that you want to happen.

The reality is that your disability insurer will be closely monitoring your bank accounts, looking for any signs that your disability is not real. They will also scrutinize your income, though that doesn't mean you can't get a dime from anywhere else. You are allowed to receive royalties linked to trademarks, books, and other such property and not be penalized for it. But if they see money coming in and interpret it as evidence that you're able to work, they can move to cut off your payments.

Your lost identity

To be sure, there is more to having a job or career than money alone. When you are no longer employed, especially if your work was a primary source of meaning in your life, you will likely experience a major identity problem. Suddenly, there will be a big gap when it comes to understanding what life is all about. If you are disabled, it is imperative that you find a means of expressing yourself to help maintain your sanity and make up for a sudden void in your life.

Short-Term and Long-Term Confusion

Extracting clear and detailed information from your employer can sometimes be frustrating.

It's not uncommon for human resource specialists to be somewhat ignorant of the ins and outs of disability. One aspect that seems more confusing than it should be relates to the differences between short-term and long-term episodes. Unfortunately, it appears that when these individuals are not up to the task or they make mistakes, ERISA and other regulations appear to make them unaccountable.

Under the circumstances, it is up to you to make sure you are informed. You should take time to learn the acronyms and terminology being used, including "PTD" – part-time disability – and "LTD – long-term disability – as well as the 'what they refer to' in different contexts.

There are often disparities between insurers and employers as to what these terms mean. Consequently, you should initiate a claim for both when you become disabled and should understand and be prepared for the requirements associated with each one. Either way, you must remember not to accept any part-time work from the moment you can no longer go to work until you have exhausted your accumulated sickness and vacation time.

Chapter 14
The COBRA Process and Options

COBRA is the abbreviation for the *Consolidated Omnibus Budget Reconciliation Act* that gives you, the now ex-worker and your family (who after leaving the workplace) the right to choose to continue Life insurance, 401(k), and group health benefits provided by their group health plan for limited periods of time, under certain circumstances such as voluntary or involuntary job loss, reduction in the hours worked, transition between jobs, disability, death, divorce, and other life events. You will be asked to pay a new qualified monthly premium for health care and life insurance coverage up to 102 % of the cost to the plan.

COBRA generally requires that group health plans sponsored by an employer with 20 or more employees in the prior year, offer employees and their families the opportunity for a temporary extension of health coverage (called continuation coverage) in certain instances where coverage under the plan would otherwise end.

A COBRA letter sent to you in the mail will outline how you, the ex-employee or your family members may elect continuation coverage.

Your likely COBRA Elements

The benefits that employers offer may include vision, dental, and other allowances but most provide these three elements:

1. 401k Savings and Investment Account
Most people transfer these funds to an individual account at their favorite financial company, such as Vanguard.

2. Medical Health Plan
Most disabled people are automatically awarded Medicare when their disability is awarded.

3. Life Insurance
Some people will sell their policy and use the money from the sale to pay bills or save for a rainy day.

Chapter 15
Selling Your Life Insurance

Once you leave work, you will get a COBRA letter that explains how you can continue your life insurance as an individual policy and then begin to pay the monthly premium out of your own bank account. Naturally, those payments are likely to be too high for you to maintain the policy.

AIG Direct, United of Omaha, Federal Trust, Fidelity Life, and American National Aetna are examples of a few of the major life insurance companies that provide plans through employers and businesses. This chapter is not singling out any of these companies but rather discusses them in a generic way. Almost all these insurance providers get customer reviews of FIVE out of FIVE stars. However, if you choose to sell your policy, there will be slow and bundling practices that delay authorization final sale.

Companies like **Coventry Direct,** educate consumers about the option to sell their life insurance policy through a life settlement, giving policy owners the choice to sell their unneeded life insurance and realize more value than a surrender or lapse.

Once you leave work, you will have a serious decision to make. That decision will be if you should convert your employer's group life insurance into a personal policy or not. The decision is yours. You may not have a spouse or children who are expecting life Insurance policy payment upon your death.

85

When you elected these life insurance plans at the old workplace, your employer took out a premium payment from your pay. The amount of your monthly deduction may be relatively small. Twenty dollars for the life insurance and one dollar and twenty-five cents a month for accident and dismemberment policy. These payments were made to the insurance companies involved with your group plan. As an example, let's say that your yearly gross in your career was $80,000.00 a year. And your group life plan paid $160,000.000 under a normal death and $240,000.00 if the death occurred while the employee was on a business trip.

Now that you are disabled, you can convert this policy to an individual plan but the monthly premium might be over 1,000.00 a month. For someone on a fixed income, this will be a large and difficult bill to pay each month.

Chapter 16
An Inspector Calls

One clear June morning, the phone rang. Gloria answered it. "Gloria Carter speaking!"

"This is Ken Cohen from United Causality Disability. I'm calling to schedule a home visit at your earliest convenience. I'd just like to ask you a few survey questions to validate your ongoing disability claim."

"Oh, okay." Her palms were beginning to sweat. "Do I need to have someone here?"

"If you want to arrange representation, that is fine," Ken said.

"I would prefer that." Her pulse began to pound in her ears. Was she right to feel nervous? Could you disqualify for disability even after you'd qualified? "Is this a routine procedure?"

"How is ten in the morning on Tuesday, August twelfth?"

"That would be fine." Panic ballooned in her stomach.

"Perfect. I'll make a note. Have a pleasant day."

After ending the call, Gloria phoned her legal advisor. "Jeff? An inspector called me from the insurance company. He's coming here to evaluate my claim. Is this a normal procedure? Am I in danger of losing my coverage? What's going to happen to me?"

"Take a breath, Gloria," Jeff said, with a reassuring chuckle. "If they're coming to your home, they will be looking to settle."

"Settle?"

"They want to get you off their payroll. We don't suggest you agree to that. If you get even ten percent of the entire payout, you'll be lucky."

"I can't deal with this. I feel like I'm in over my head."

"That's what I'm here for. I'll take care of this for you."

"Oh my God. Thank you! I need your help."

"I'll be right there with you. We'll make a little plan. After twenty minutes or so, I will ask you if you're getting tired. You'll say yes, and I'll get him out the door and send him on his way. There is nothing new to report."

Gloria's shoulders relaxed. "That sounds fine. All right then."

Two days later, Gloria received a letter by Federal Express mail.

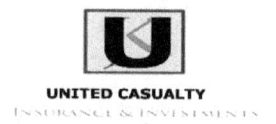

UNITED CASUALTY
INSURANCE & INVESTMENTS

1 5 9 856
info@jackson......om
www.jacks...kennedy.com
P.O. Box 3 3, hill street, NY

Dear Ms. Carter,

This is to confirm our appointment at your home on Tuesday, August 12th. I will take you through a survey and record your answers, and you will need to sign off on this afterward. I will record our discussion using a computer.

Kenneth Cohen
Casualty Insurance Investigator

On Tuesday morning, at ten o'clock sharp, the doorbell rang. Jeff went downstairs to answer it. Gloria was propped up in her bed with two chairs angled toward her.

Jeff guided Ken into the bedroom.

"Nice to meet you, Gloria. I'm Ken. We spoke on the phone, remember?"

"Of course, I do," Gloria said.

"Right, so as I explained in my letter, I'll be guiding you through a short survey." He cleared his throat. "Say, could I trouble you for a glass of water?"

"I'll get it," Jeff said and left the room.

Ken swiftly approached the bed and loomed over Gloria. "So, how are we feeling?" He arched an eyebrow. "A bit up and down, I see? Good days and bad days, mmm?" His teeth were very white.

Gloria swallowed hard. "Excuse me?"

"Some good days and some bad."

"Um, no—every day is the same. They are all bad." Feeling a sudden pain in her neck, she tried to massage it away.

Jeff returned with a glass of water and handed it to Ken, who set it on the nightstand without taking a sip. They sat in the chairs facing Gloria's bed. Ken opened his laptop. As it powered up, he settled back in his chair. "Can I ask you a few questions?"

"Of course." Gloria smiled.

"Are you able to dress yourself every day?"

"Yes, I can."

He typed something on the laptop. "Can you do housework?"

Gloria shook her head. "I hire someone to come in and take care of that. They wash the dishes and organize the cupboards."

"Are you able to walk to and from the store and any other places?"

"My strength is limited. My grocer is a few hundred yards away; so I can just about make it there when I need to."

He entered a keystroke with a loud *click.* "One more thing—who is Marla Parks?"

The hair on her arms stood on end. There would be no point in lying, as he already knew the truth. "He—I mean Marla Parks—doesn't exist. I mean, it's a pen name."

Jeff's eyebrows shot up. He looked at Gloria. Gloria looked at Jeff and then turned away.

Ken feigned dramatic surprise. "A pen name? Wow. Am I to understand—are you an author?" He pronounced the word *author* as if it were the name of a poisonous creature.

Gloria shrugged. "I've written an e-book, yes. It only sold a few hundred copies."

"I see," Ken said, looking pleased with himself. "So, in fact, Marla *does* exist. Nice to meet you, Marla."

"I don't see—I mean, I declared my earnings and filed everything in my yearly taxes."

"Whoa," Jeff interjected, "you might not want to bring up the subject of taxes."

"Too late," Gloria said, with a bitter laugh.

Ken continued with his line of questioning. "Are you able to prepare meals for yourself?"

"I can't cook anything. I can assemble a salad, and that's about it. If I want a hot meal, I have to get something delivered."

"Are you taking all the medications prescribed by your doctor?"

"Yes. Although they often make me feel fatigued," she said, casting Jeff a meaningful glance.

Jeff recognized his cue. "Are you okay, Gloria? Getting tired?"

Gloria nodded. "I'm fading."

Ken clicked a few keys. "Fine, I won't keep you any longer." He stood up and approached the bed, holding out the laptop and a stylus. "I just need your signature right here. I can print it off back at the office and send you a copy. Here. Just sign directly on the screen."

Jeff crossed the room. "Let me read it first."

Ken handed him the laptop. "Sure."

Jeff skimmed the screen before handing the laptop to Gloria, who signed and handed the laptop and stylus back to Jeff.

Jeff smiled reassuringly as he tucked everything away. He looked at Jeff, "If I need anything else, I'll contact you to schedule another appointment. I hope you get adjusted to your medications and start to feel much better."

"Thank you," Gloria said.

Jeff shook Ken's hand and escorted him out. As the two men walked down the stairs, Gloria could hear Jeff's voice echoing in the landing. "I know you'll do everything in your power to expedite this process. I'll be following your every move very closely, so I'll always be up to speed and can assist wherever needed. I've handled a lot of cases and I know the protocol."

Gloria's eyes widened in surprise. She'd never known Jeff could be so subtly forceful and intimidating. Perhaps everything was going to be fine. Still, when Jeff returned, she recounted to him Ken's peculiar "good days and bad days" comment.

Two weeks later, the insurance company requested Gloria's tax records, going back six years. She quickly complied, collating them and forwarding them to Jeff to send to the insurer. Gloria has continued to receive regular payments from the insurer and has received no further requests, nor encountered any interference. She is free!

Chapter 17
What's Next Financially

This is the time to be completely honest with yourself. In the morning ask yourself, "What are the things you have always disliked and wanted to improve?" Such as not spend so much time on mindless TV shows or video games each day. These are small secrets you've kept to yourself, like hygiene habits, talking habits and so on. Let's say, you always arrive late for any and all appointments. It is a nagging habit. Well, this might be the time to fix this little character flaw. When you worked day in and day out, you probably stacked these flaws up and ignored them for the time. But now is the time. It is your time. Imagine if you could repair a few flaws you have been carrying around as baggage, how wonderful and light you'd feel.

Downsizing

Many disabled people will downsize their excess belongings and accumulations. Eliminating extra mobile phones, magazine subscriptions, internet subscriptions, cable TV's, and all sorts of old memories are a necessity. Look for all those things that are not worth moving, donating, or even conferring about: old spices, junk mail, old magazines (yes, even all those yellow-spine NATIONAL GEOGRAPHIC issues), outdated medications, unused toiletries, plastic food containers, candles, stuffed toys (most charities won't accept them), and the contents of the junk drawer (just hang onto change and spare keys).

If you own a high-maintenance home with a large yard that requires upkeep, consider selling the property and renting a smaller apartment or mobile home.

Planning Your Financial Future

The next step is to look at a broader plan of action for growing whatever is left of your wealth, which can be loosely set forth as follows:

Grow-Your-Wealth-Plan

1. Live within the constraints of your budget.
2. Limit your use of credit.
3. Purchase assets that can compound or grow in value over time.

Needless to say, this simple approach is at odds with what you may have long been doing before your disability. You may not need fancy cars, luxury, apparel and expensive vacations; or to rely on credit to acquire those things you can no longer afford. It is a topsy-turvy world where debt is not the prison that limits our choices and money is seen as something other than powerful.

Budget

None of us likes to budget, but now, you must. Use your natural power of intention and become frugal. You need to gain control of such emotions and habits of spending, and count your money, not in dollars, but pennies.

An effective, balanced budget begins with knowledge. You need to understand your spending habits and figure out which expenditures are necessary and which aren't. Do you know where your money goes each day? If not, then it's time to start keeping track with a simple diary of your daily expenditures.

To begin with, you'll need to wade through your bank statements, starting with the most recent month. Write down how much you spend on rent, utilities, food, insurance and other necessities. Move on to the credit and loans you regularly pay down. Finally, dive in and look at everything else, especially the little stuff. Don't forget to include items you purchase with a credit card or payments that are automatically deducted from your bank and other financial accounts.

Over the next several weeks and months, set aside a few moments each day to track your spending habits. That's right, make a habit of tracking your spending habits. It's best to find a time when you have a little creative energy. Some of us are morning people; others like to burn their creative juices later in the evening. Whatever the case, make sure you can remain focused on this activity; it is one that is necessary for you to achieve your financial budget.

To initiate your daily routine, place a blank sheet of paper on your desk or use the worksheet document on a computer. Then try to recall the day's purchases or use your bank receipts. Did you buy coffee, breakfast or milk for the children? Do you remember how much you had in your wallet or pocket to begin with? Did you tip someone? Ask yourself plenty of questions. You don't need to record exact amounts--you can use approximate values, when necessary--but try to avoid low-ball estimates.

The next step is to list your regular monthly payments and arrange them in order of priority. Monthly payments might be collected from your bank account. Then, based on the daily cash spending lists, you can get a monthly idea of where your money goes. Although the list will vary depending upon your individual needs and circumstances, the end result will probably look something like this:

_____Payment to your investment fund
_____Rent/Mortgage
_____Car Payments
_____Medical Insurance
_____Dental and Vision Insurance
_____Medications
_____Car Insurance
_____Car Gas and Maintenance
_____Car Parking, Tickets and Tolls
_____Home Insurance
_____Groceries
_____Laundry and Dry Cleaning
_____Phone
_____Gas and Electricity
_____Cable Television
_____Internet
_____Entertainment Movies, Theater
_____Entertainment, Outings, Dinners
_____Credit card 1
_____Credit card 2
_____Other

Set your budget and stick with it by placing it in front of you every day. Leave it on your desk so you are reminded to record all historical spending splurges.

Potential Money Savers

1. Reduce gift purchases on special holidays such as Valentine's Day, Flower Day and Christmas. Being with someone and enjoying their company or a call to someone special is free and personal.
2. Instead of buying books and magazines, why not use the resources that are freely available on the internet.
3. Get a library card; books, movies and CDs and even internet time are usually completely free.

4. Watch out for regular, recurring charges from Amazon Prime and Spotify.
5. The daily newspaper: If you can't get by without having a physical newspaper, why not share the cost of the purchase with a friend?
6. Studies have shown that, in most cases, bottled water is not really better for you than the stuff that comes from a tap. Why not go for the latter?
7. It's no fun being cold, but it might be better for your financial future if you keep the thermostat turned down and wear layers and sweaters instead. Winter time: You might also want to consider closing off the rooms you don't use to save even more on your heating bills.
8. Try to eliminate all those unhealthy pleasures and empty calories that are draining your pockets. Cigarettes, tea, soda, cigars, alcohol, candy, donuts, and wine can be very costly--in more ways than one, especially over the long term.
9. It is one of life's daily staples, but coffee can be quite an expensive habit. Eliminate or cut your consumption in half. Stop going to the expensive shops--is their brand really *that* much better? Instead, stretch your budget with instant coffee and store label varieties, or maybe even switch to pure hot water.
10. Take a close look at all the other things in your life that once seemed like must-haves but are no longer necessary. Cancel the book clubs and Sports Illustrated magazine subscription and start thinking about whether you really need to own all those high-end clothes and accessories.
11. If you can't live without seeing those big-time sporting events, how about booking the cheap seats and inviting some friends along to enjoy the fun? It will be a blast! If you pay for NFL Sunday Ticket, share the cost by having friends over who can pitch in on the fee or bring all the food.

12. Auto insurance is another expense that most of us can't do without. But that doesn't mean there's nothing you can do about it. Shop around for other quotes or contact your insurance agent to see if you can prudently reduce your existing coverage, raise your deductibles or eliminate certain options, such as towing and loss of use, which you probably don't need anyway.
13. Ask for discounts wherever you go. Just because a retailer has a price listed on that pair of pants or something else you might need to buy, that doesn't mean you can't get it cheaper, especially if you make it clear that you might have to take your business elsewhere.
14. Rethinking the way you handle your day-to-day banking needs can also pay dividends. You are charged a fee when you withdraw money from ATMs that are not associated with your financial institution, often by the ATM owner *and* your bank. Those small charges can really add up. If you can't use an in-network machine, try to find one with a low fee or get extra cash back with your debit card when you buy that instant coffee at the grocery store.
15. Don't forget about the other fees that banks charge. You might be able to save at least a hundred dollars or more a year by keeping a higher balance in your account than you do now. If not, maybe you should think about switching to an institution offering a better deal. You should also avoid bouncing checks or be using nonessential services. Banks make a lot of money from the fees they charge; don't let them profit at your expense.
16. Telephone chargers and computers left plugged in 24 hours a day are costly. Large screen TVs use excessive power.
17. Last but not least, remember to ask questions of yourself and others. People are always finding a

better deal or a way to save. Tapping the wisdom of friends, co-workers and internet social networks can be a great way to make sure you spend less and have more!

Chapter 18
Finding Meaning and Purpose

I hope that, before too long, the maelstrom of thunder storms will have stopped spinning around you and, with the help of your doctor, your life coach, and your lawyer, you will have landed on solid ground. Expectantly, the thunderstorm has calmed and your sight of the future is becoming clear. With any luck the mental burdens have recessed. You may feel somewhat battered, and a little frayed around the edges, but you are alive. The treacherous journey hasn't destroyed you—it has strengthened your resolve and your confidence. You, my friend, are a survivor.

Your new journey does not have to entail suffering, as long as you hold yourself responsible for defining meaning and purpose in your life. Each individual is unique. Your dreams will manifest inside you and guide you towards your life's purpose. Here are some ways in which you might wish to express yourself and connect with those around you, in order to encourage your individual passions to come to life.

Love, and be loved in return

- Spend time with someone you love.
- Babysit the children of friends or relatives.
- Take care of a sick or older relative.
- Tutor a close friend or relative.
- Homeschool a relative's child or children.

Connect socially

- Adopt a pet.

- Smile and say hello to those you encounter during your daily walk.
- Invite someone out for coffee or to a sporting event.
- Volunteer at church groups, fraternal activities, youth clubs, and sports programs.
- Help out at your local soup kitchen or other community outreach project.

Communicate with others

- Write and publish a book.
- Start a blog.
- Create YouTube videos.

Offer your skills

- Repair electrical gadgets or cars, for family and friends.

Conclusion

You have the time and will to think beyond the threats to yourself and reach out to others and serve something greater than yourself in a meaningful way that matches your situation. Certain sayings are repeated and become cliché because they are true. Life is worth living and this moment in time may be your finest hour. Seize each day and make it extraordinary by manifesting your absolute best.

The End

CPSIA information can be obtained
at www.ICGtesting.com
Printed in the USA
LVHW081329071019
633420LV00012B/504/P